MORNING PILATES FOR BEGINNERS

Rise and Align with Pilates as starters

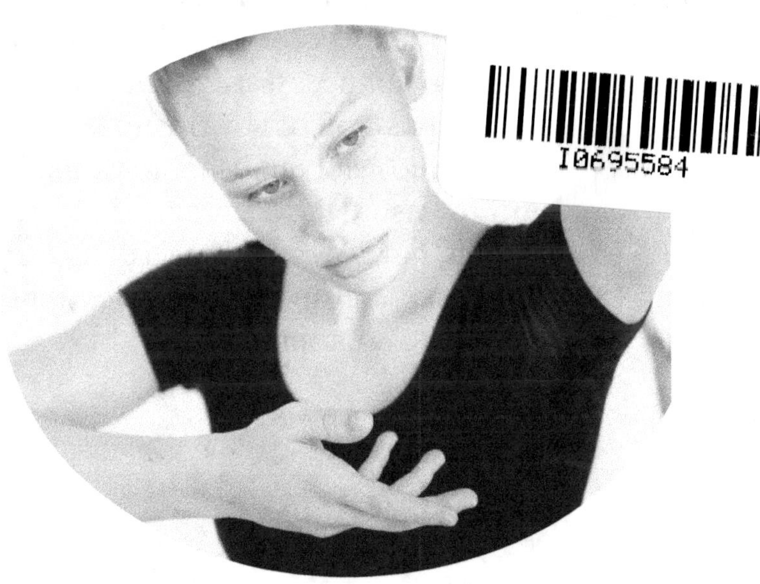

Lawrence R. Hale

Table of contents

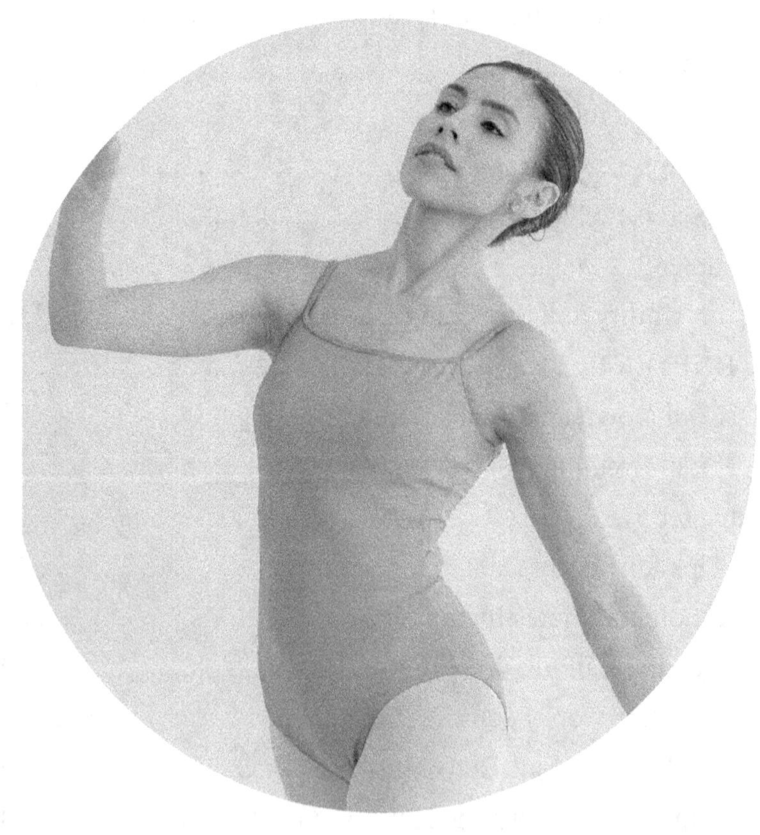

INTRODUCTION

Welcome to Morning Pilates for Beginners

Welcome to the world of Morning Pilates, a gentle and invigorating way to start your day with renewed energy and a refreshed mind. Whether you're new to Pilates or looking for a gentle morning routine to kick start your day, this guide is designed to help you embark on a journey of physical well-being and self-discovery.

Benefits of Morning Pilates

Morning Pilates offers a multitude of benefits that extend beyond the physical realm. As you engage in these mindful movements and controlled exercises, you'll experience:

Improved Flexibility: Pilates emphasizes stretching and lengthening muscles, helping you increase your flexibility over time. This newfound flexibility can make daily movements more comfortable and reduce the risk of injury.

Enhanced Core Strength: Core strength is at the heart of Pilates. By targeting the muscles that support your spine and pelvis, you'll not only achieve a toned midsection but also develop better posture and stability.

Stress Reduction: The deliberate focus on breathing and controlled movements in Pilates can have a calming effect on your nervous system. This can help reduce stress and anxiety, leaving you feeling more centered and focused for the day ahead.

Increased Body Awareness: Morning Pilates encourages mindfulness of your body and its movements. You'll become more in tune with how your body feels, functions, and responds to various exercises, fostering a deeper connection between your body and mind.

Low Impact, High Rewards: Unlike some high-impact workouts, Pilates is gentle on the joints, making it suitable for individuals of all fitness levels. It's an excellent choice for beginners and those with limited exercise experience.

Safety Precautions

Before you embark on your Morning Pilates journey, it's essential to consider some safety precautions:

Consult Your Healthcare Provider: If you have any medical conditions, injuries, or concerns about your fitness level, it's advisable to consult your healthcare provider or a qualified fitness professional before starting any exercise program.

Listen to Your Body: Throughout your Pilates practice, always pay attention to how your body feels. If you experience pain or discomfort, modify the exercises or skip them altogether. It's crucial to work within your comfort zone and gradually progress.

Stay Hydrated: Hydration is essential for any exercise routine. Make sure to drink water before and after your session to keep your body adequately fueled.

Use Proper Form: Proper form is key to the effectiveness of Pilates exercises and minimizing the risk of injury. This guide will provide detailed instructions on form for each exercise.

Be Patient: Pilates is about progress, not perfection. It may take time to build strength and flexibility, so be patient with yourself and celebrate your achievements along the way.

As you embark on this journey, remember that Morning Pilates is not just a physical exercise routine; it's an opportunity to nurture your well-being holistically. Therefore by dedicating time to your body and mind each morning, you're setting the tone for a productive and balanced day ahead. So, let's get started on this empowering and rejuvenating path to a healthier you!

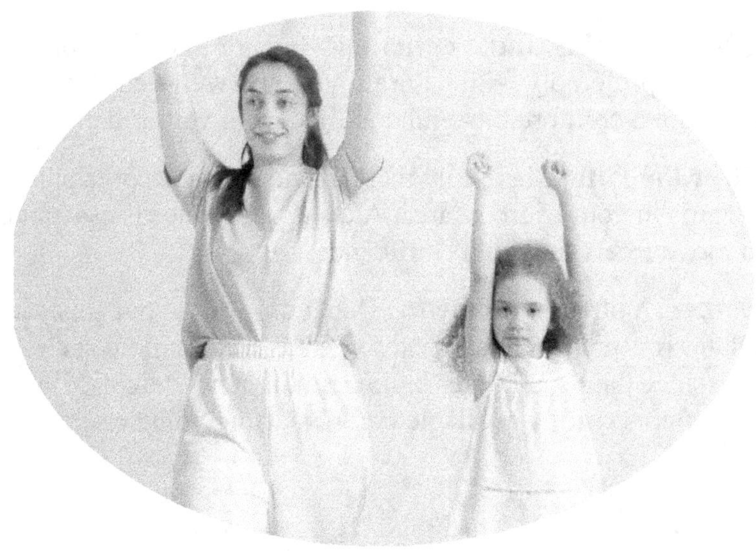

Chapter 1

Getting Started

Setting up Your Space

Before you begin your Morning Pilates routine, it's essential to create an environment that promotes focus, comfort, and safety. Learn how to set up your space effectively bellow

Designate a Quiet Area: Choose a quiet, clutter-free area in your home where you can practice without distractions. This space can be a corner of your living room, a spare room, or any area where you feel comfortable.

Use a Yoga Mat: A yoga or Pilates mat provides a cushioned and non-slip surface for your exercises. It's crucial for comfort and preventing injuries.

Check Lighting and Ventilation: Ensure that the room is well-lit, preferably with natural light, and well-ventilated to maintain a comfortable temperature during your practice.

Clear the Path: Make sure there are no obstacles or tripping hazards in your exercise area. A clear, safe space is essential to move freely and with confidence.

Gather Your Equipment: Depending on your chosen Pilates routine, you may need some basic equipment such as resistance bands, a Pilates ball, or small hand weights. Have these items readily available before starting your session.

Choosing the Right Attire

Selecting appropriate attire for your Morning Pilates session can significantly enhance your experience:

Comfort is Key: Choose comfortable, form-fitting clothing that allows you to move freely without restrictions. Avoid baggy attire that may get in the way during exercises.

Footwear: Most Pilates exercises are done barefoot, but you can wear non-slip socks with grip if you prefer. These can provide added stability during certain movements.

Layers: If you're practicing in a cooler environment, consider layering your clothing, so you can remove layers as you warm up.

Equipment You May Need

While many Pilates exercises can be done with just your body weight, some routines incorporate equipment to add variety and resistance. Here's an overview of common Pilates equipment:

Pilates Mat: As mentioned earlier, a comfortable mat provides a supportive surface for your exercises. It's especially useful for floor work.

Resistance Bands: These elastic bands come in various strengths and can be used to add resistance to your exercises, helping you build strength and tone muscles.

Pilates Ball: A small inflatable ball can be used for added support and stability during specific exercises, particularly for targeting the core and improving balance.

Small Hand Weights: While not necessary for beginners, small hand weights can be incorporated into advanced Pilates routines to increase the challenge.

Pilates Reformer: Reformer machines are common in Pilates studios but may not be accessible for everyone. These machines offer a wide range of exercises and resistance options. If you have access to a reformer and are interested in using it, consult with a certified Pilates instructor for guidance.

Now that you've set up your space, chosen the right attire, and gathered any necessary equipment, you're ready to embark on your Morning Pilates journey. **Chapter 2** will guide you through essential warm-up exercises to prepare your body for the practice ahead. Always remember that the key to success in Pilates is consistency and patience. By taking these initial steps, you're setting yourself up for a rewarding and transformative experience in the world of

Core Exercises

Core strength is the foundation of Pilates, and this chapter will introduce you to a series of core-focused exercises designed to strengthen and stabilize your abdominal muscles, lower back, and pelvic area. As a beginner, building a strong core is essential for maintaining proper posture, improving balance, and preventing injuries.

The Pilates Hundred

The Pilates Hundred is a classic exercise that not only challenges your core but also helps you focus on your breath and control. Here's how to perform it:

Starting Position:

Lie on your back on the mat with your legs extended and arms by your sides. Lift up your legs away from the ground, knees bent at a ninety degree angle. Engage your abdominal muscles, pressing your lower back into the mat.

Exercise:

Inhale deeply through your nose for a count of five as you pump your arms up and down by your sides.

Exhale completely through your mouth for a count of five as you continue pumping your arms.

Maintain a strong core, and keep your gaze toward your knees. Continue this pattern for a total of 100 arm pumps (hence the name).

The Pilates Hundred is an excellent exercise for warming up your core and increasing your heart rate, making it an ideal choice for the beginning of your Pilates routine.

Leg Raises

Leg raises target your lower abdominal muscles, helping to tone and strengthen your core. Here's how to do them:

Starting Position:

Your arms should be by your sides as you lay on your back with your legs extended. Keep your lower back pressed into the mat to engage your core.

Exercise:

Inhale as you slowly raise your legs off the ground, keeping them straight.

Exhale as you lower your legs back down without letting them touch the mat.

Repeat for a predetermined number of reps, progressively increasing as your strength improves.

Plank Variations

Planks are exceptional for strengthening your entire core, including your abdominal muscles, obliques, and lower back below are some planks variants that you can experiment with: Traditional

Plank: Start in a push-up position with your hands directly under your shoulders. Keep your body in a straight line from head to heels, engaging your core.

Hold this position for as long as you can, aiming to increase your time with each session.

Side Plank:

Stack your legs on top of one other and lie on your side. Keep your elbow directly beneath your shoulder. Lift your hips off the ground to form a straight line from your head to your heels. Hold this position, then switch to the other side.

Pilates Roll-Up

The Pilates Roll-Up is a classic exercise for building strength in your core and improving flexibility in your spine. Here's how to do it:

Starting Position:

Lie on your back with your legs outstretched and your arms spread overhead.

Exercise:

Inhale as you lift your arms toward the ceiling and begin to roll up, reaching for your toes.

Exhale as you continue to reach forward, moving your spine sequentially off the mat.

Roll back down one vertebra at a time, keeping your core engaged.

Repeat for a set number of repetitions.

Bridges

Bridges work your glutes, lower back, and core. They also help improve hip mobility and strengthen the posterior chain. Here's how to perform them:

Starting Position:

Lie flat on your back with your knees bent and your feet hip-width apart. Position your arms at your sides, palms down.

.

Exercise:

Inhale as you press through your heels and lift your hips off the ground, creating a straight line from your shoulders to your knees.

You will squeeze your glutes at the top of the movement .Exhale as you lower your hips back down. Repeat for a set number of repetitions.

These core exercises are fundamental in developing a strong foundation for your Pilates practice. As a beginner, focus on mastering the form and gradually increasing the number of repetitions or duration for each exercise. Core strength is not only beneficial for your Pilates practice but also for daily activities and overall posture. In **Chapter 3**, we'll explore flexibility and stretching exercises to enhance your body's range of motion and balance

Flexibility and Stretching

Flexibility and stretching exercises are vital components of any Pilates routine, helping to improve your range of motion, reduce the risk of injury, and enhance overall body balance. In this chapter, we'll explore various stretches and flexibility exercises that are suitable for beginners.

Spine Stretch Forward (Saw)

The Spine Stretch Forward, also known as the Saw, is a seated Pilates exercise that promotes spinal flexibility, stretches the hamstrings, and engages the core. Here's how to perform it:

Starting Position:

Sit tall on your mat with your legs extended in front of you, hip-width apart. Flex your feet, and then you will engage your core muscles.

Exercise:

Inhale to lengthen your spine and sit up tall. Exhale as you rotate your upper body to the right, reaching your left hand toward your right foot.

Imagine sawing off your pinky toe with your right hand while keeping your spine straight.

Inhale to return to the center, then exhale as you rotate to the left, reaching your right hand toward your left foot.

Repeat this sawing motion for a set number of repetitions.

The Saw is an excellent exercise for improving spinal mobility, enhancing the flexibility of your hamstrings, and strengthening your core muscles.

Butterfly Stretch

The Butterfly Stretch is a seated stretch that targets the inner thighs and groin muscles. It's a gentle exercise that promotes flexibility in the hips and can be modified for varying levels of flexibility:

Starting Position:

Sit on your mat with your knees bent and the soles of your feet together.

Hold onto your ankles with your hands.

Exercise:

Inhale as you lengthen your spine, sitting up tall.

Exhale as you gently press your knees toward the ground, using your elbows.

Hold the stretch for a few deep breaths, feeling a gentle stretch in your inner thighs.

If comfortable, you can increase the stretch by leaning your torso forward slightly.

The Butterfly Stretch is an excellent way to improve hip flexibility and alleviate tension in the inner thigh area.

Seated Twist

The Seated Twist is a seated Pilates exercise that provides a deep stretch for the spine and helps improve spinal mobility. Here's how to perform it:

Starting Position:

Sit with your legs stretched in front of you on your mat. Place your right foot flat on the ground after crossing it over your left leg. Put your left elbow outside your right knee.

Exercise: Inhale in other to elongate your spine, sitting up tall.

Exhale as you gently twist your torso to the right, using your left elbow to deepen the stretch.

Keep your gaze over your right shoulder and hold the stretch for a few deep breaths.

Inhale to return to the center, then repeat on the other side.

The Seated Twist is an effective exercise for improving spinal flexibility and releasing tension in the back muscles.

Hamstring Stretch

The Hamstring Stretch is crucial for enhancing the flexibility of your hamstrings and can be performed in various ways. Here's a seated version for beginners:

Starting Position:

Sit on your mat with your legs extended in front of you, keeping your feet flexed.

Exercise:

Inhale to elongate your spine, while sitting up tall.

Exhale as you hinge at your hips and reach your hands toward your toes.

Keep your back straight, and only go as far as you can while maintaining a comfortable stretch.

Hold the stretch for a few deep breaths, feeling the stretch in your hamstrings.

The Hamstring Stretch is essential for improving leg flexibility and can be incorporated into your routine to increase mobility and reduce the risk of muscle tightness.

Cool Down

After completing your flexibility and stretching exercises, it's essential to incorporate a cool-down period to relax your muscles and bring your heart rate back to its resting state. This phase can include gentle stretches or relaxation techniques like deep breathing exercises and the Corpse Pose (Savasana).

The Corpse Pose, also known as Savasana, involves lying on your back with your arms and legs extended, palms facing up. Close your eyes, relax your entire body, and focus on your breath. Allow yourself to release any tension and find a sense of tranquility. Savasana is a time for reflection and a perfect way to conclude your Morning Pilates routine, leaving you feeling refreshed and balanced.

Incorporating flexibility and stretching exercises into your Pilates routine is essential for maintaining a healthy range of motion, preventing muscle imbalances, and promoting relaxation. These exercises can be customized to suit your individual needs and can be gradually advanced as you progress in your Pilates practice. In Chapter 5, we will explore cool-down and relaxation techniques to conclude your Morning Pilates routine effectively.

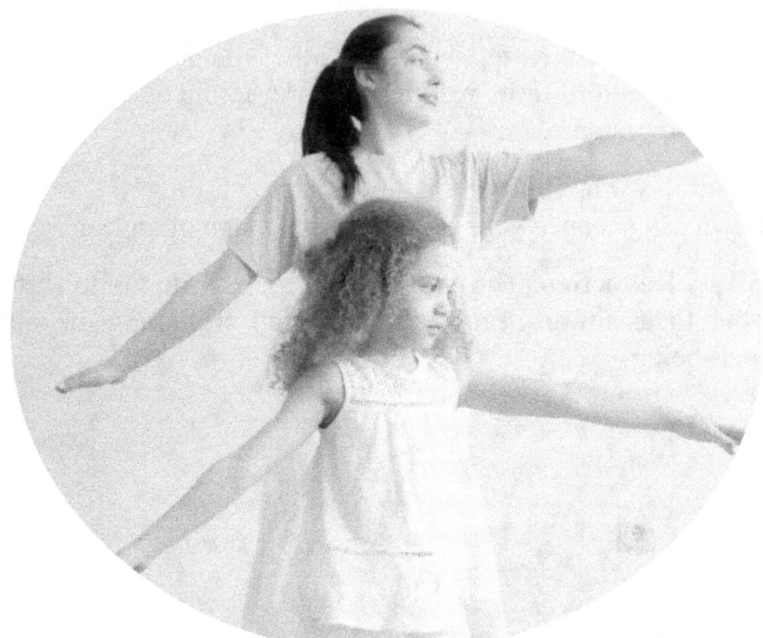

CHAPTER 4

Cool Down and Relaxation

As you near the end of your Morning Pilates session, it's crucial to transition from the active exercises into a state of relaxation and calm. This chapter will guide you through the cool-down phase and relaxation techniques that promote recovery and mental clarity.

Importance of Cooling Down

The cool-down phase is often overlooked, but it's a vital part of your Pilates practice. Here's why it matters:

Muscle Recovery: Cooling down helps your muscles recover from the exertion of the exercises. It reduces the risk of post-workout soreness and stiffness.

Gradual Heart Rate Decline: It allows your heart rate to gradually return to its resting rate, preventing abrupt drops in blood pressure.

Promotes Flexibility: Gentle stretches during the cool-down can enhance your flexibility and range of motion.

Stress Reduction: The cool-down is an opportunity to shift your focus inward, reducing stress and promoting mental well-being.

Before moving into static stretches, start with deep breathing exercises to calm your mind and bring your body into a state of relaxation.

Diaphragmatic Breathing:

Place one hand on your chest and the other on your belly while lying on your back.

Deeply inhale through your nose, allowing your belly to rise while your chest remains stationary.

Slowly exhale through your lips, feeling your abdomen drop. Continue this deep breathing pattern for a few minutes, focusing on the rise and fall of your abdomen.

Static Stretches

After deep breathing exercises, transition into static stretches to target specific muscle groups.

Child's Pose:

Begin in a kneeling position.

Sit back on your heels with your arms stretched out on the mat..

Rest your forehead on the ground.

Hold for 30 seconds to 1 minute, focusing on deep breaths.

Cat-Cow Stretch:

Come to a tabletop position with your hands under your shoulders and knees under your hips.

Inhale while arching your back and elevating your head and tailbone into Cow Pose.

Exhale as you circle your back (Cat Pose), tucking your chin and tailbone.

Flow between Cat and Cow for 1-2 minutes, syncing your breath with the movements.

Seated Forward Bend:

Sit with your legs outstretched in front of you.

Inhale to lengthen your spine.

Exhale as you tilt at the hips and reach towards your toes.

Hold for 30 seconds to 1 minute, keeping your back straight and breathing deeply.

Savasana (Corpse Pose)

The Savasana, also known as the Corpse Pose, is a classic yoga and Pilates relaxation pose that brings your practice to a peaceful conclusion.

Starting Position:

Lie on your back on your mat with your legs extended and arms by your sides, palms facing up.

Exercise:

Take a few long breaths to settle into the position.

Relax your entire body, beginning with your toes and working your way up to your head.

Let go of any tension, allowing your body to feel heavy and supported by the mat.

Clear your mind and focus on your breath. Inhale and exhale slowly and deeply.

Remain in Savasana for 5-10 minutes or as long as you like, experiencing a sense of deep relaxation and mental clarity.

Savasana is a profound way to conclude your Morning Pilates routine. It allows your body and mind to fully absorb the benefits of your practice, leaving you with a sense of rejuvenation and inner peace. It's a time to reflect on your efforts and appreciate the physical and mental growth you've achieved.

As you integrate cool-down and relaxation techniques into your Morning Pilates routine, remember that consistency is key. This chapter serves as a reminder that your Pilates practice is not just about physical fitness but also about nurturing your mental and emotional well-being. By dedicating time to relaxation and self-care, you're setting the tone for a balanced and harmonious day ahead.

Chapter 5

Tips for Success

Achieving success in your Morning Pilates routine involves more than just following exercises. It's about creating a sustainable and fulfilling practice that supports your well-being. This chapter provides valuable insights and tips to help you make the most of your Pilates journey.

Staying Consistent

Consistency is the key to reaping the benefits of Pilates. Here's how to maintain a consistent practice:

Set a Schedule: Dedicate specific days and times for your Morning Pilates sessions. Consistency is easier to achieve with a structured routine.

Start Slowly: If you're new to exercise, begin with shorter sessions and gradually increase the duration and intensity as your fitness level improves.

Accountability: Share your Pilates goals with a friend or family member who can help keep you accountable.

Variety: Keep your practice engaging by exploring different Pilates routines and exercises. Variety prevents boredom and plateaus.

Listening to Your Body

Paying attention to your body's signals is crucial for a safe and effective Pilates practice:

Modify When Necessary: If an exercise feels too challenging or causes discomfort, don't hesitate to modify it or skip it entirely. Pilates should never be painful.

Proper Form: Focus on maintaining proper form throughout your practice. Quality trumps quantity. It's better to perform fewer repetitions with excellent form than to rush through exercises.

Rest and Recovery: Allow your body time to rest and recover between sessions. It is important to know that Overtraining can lead to burnout and injury.

Gradual Progression

As you gain experience, aim to progress gradually:

Increase Intensity: Gradually increase the intensity of your exercises by adding repetitions, resistance, or more advanced variations.

Set Goals: Define specific, achievable goals for your Pilates practice. Having clear objectives can motivate you to continue and measure your progress.

Seek Guidance: Consider working with a certified Pilates instructor as you advance. They can provide personalized guidance and help you reach your goals safely.

If you're serious about your Pilates practice, working with a qualified instructor can be immensely beneficial:

Certification Matters: Ensure your instructor is certified in Pilates. Look for qualifications from reputable organizations.

Personalized Instruction: An instructor can tailor exercises to your individual needs and provide hands-on guidance to improve your form.

Motivation and Accountability: Having an instructor can keep you motivated and accountable for your practice.

Additional Resources: In addition to classes, instructors often provide valuable resources, such as exercise plans and tips for improving your practice.

If you can adopt these tips into your Morning Pilates routine, you'll set yourself up for a successful and fulfilling experience. Note that Pilates is not just about physical fitness but also about building a deeper connection with your body and mind. As you progress on your journey, celebrate your achievements, stay open to growth, and embrace the holistic benefits that Pilates can offer. With dedication and patience, you'll find yourself reaping the rewards of improved strength, flexibility, and overall well-being.

Congratulations on embarking on your journey into the world of Morning Pilates for beginners! As you wrap up this guide, it's essential to reflect on the knowledge you've gained and the positive changes you've experienced in your life. Morning Pilates is more than just a series of exercises; it's a path to holistic well-being, physical strength, and inner balance.

Throughout this guide, we've explored the foundations of Morning Pilates, from setting up your practice space to understanding the benefits of consistent and mindful routines. You've learned about warm-up exercises, core workouts, flexibility and stretching techniques, cooling down, and the significance of relaxation and self-care.

Pilates is not merely a physical practice; it's an opportunity to nurture your mind-body connection, develop self-awareness, and find harmony within yourself. As you continue your Morning Pilates journey, here are some key takeaways to carry with you:

Consistency is Key: Success in Pilates comes from regular practice. Commit to your routine, even on days when motivation wanes.

Ensure to listen to Your Body: Your body will always communicate its needs to you. Pay attention to any discomfort or fatigue and adapt your practice accordingly.

Progress is Personal: Embrace the journey. Your progress may be gradual, but each step forward is a victory worth celebrating.

Quality over Quantity: Focus on performing exercises with impeccable form rather than rushing through them. Precision is the essence of Pilates.

Mindful Presence: Pilates encourages mindfulness. Be present in each movement, breathe intentionally, and cultivate a deeper connection with your body.

Self-Care Matters: Pilates extends beyond physical fitness. It's an act of self-care that enhances your overall well-being, both physically and mentally.

Instructor Guidance: If you're eager to take your practice to the next level, consider working with a certified Pilates instructor. They are in the position to provide you with expert guidance and personalized instruction.

As you continue your Morning Pilates practice, remember that each session is an opportunity to grow, learn, and strengthen not only your body but also your mind and spirit. The benefits extend far beyond the mat, influencing how you navigate daily challenges and approach life with a sense of balance and vitality.

Whether you're seeking increased flexibility, improved core strength, stress reduction, or a gentle start to your day, Morning Pilates has something to offer you. It's a practice that empowers you to take charge of your well-being and invest in your health and happiness.

So, as you roll up your mat and carry the lessons of this guide with you into your daily life, remember that Morning Pilates is not just a physical routine; it's a journey of self-discovery, resilience, and transformation. Embrace it with an open heart, and may your mornings be filled with vitality, balance, and a deep sense of inner peace. Here's to your continued success in your Morning Pilates journey!

Appendix: Sample Weekly Routine

Creating a structured weekly routine can help you stay committed to your Morning Pilates practice. Below, you'll find a sample weekly routine that you can use as a starting point. Feel free to adjust it based on your goals, fitness level, and time availability.

Monday: Core Focus

Warm-Up: Gentle neck stretches, shoulder rolls, Cat-Cow stretch (5 minutes)

Core Exercises: The Pilates Hundred, Leg Raises, and Plank Variations (15-20 minutes)

Flexibility: Spine Stretch Forward, Butterfly Stretch (5 minutes)

Cool Down: Savasana (Corpse Pose) (5 minutes)

Wednesday: Full-Body Workout

Warm-Up: Gentle neck stretches, shoulder rolls, Cat-Cow stretch (5 minutes)

Full-Body Exercises: Pilates Roll-Up, Bridges, Side Leg Lifts (15-20 minutes)

Flexibility: Seated Twist, Hamstring Stretch (5 minutes)

Cool Down: Savasana (Corpse Pose) (5 minutes)

Friday: Flexibility and Relaxation

Warm-Up: Gentle neck stretches, shoulder rolls, Cat-Cow stretch (5 minutes)

Flexibility: Spine Stretch Forward, Butterfly Stretch, Seated Forward Bend (15-20 minutes)

Cool Down and Relaxation: Deep breathing exercises, Savasana (Corpse Pose) (10 minutes)

Appendix: Glossary

Below are key terms and phrases frequently used in Pilates that you may encounter during your practice

Core: The muscles of the abdomen, lower back, and pelvic region, which provide stability and support for the spine and pelvis.

Pilates Mat: A specialized mat designed for Pilates exercises, providing cushioning and a non-slip surface.

Resistance Bands: Elastic bands used to add resistance to Pilates exercises, helping to strengthen and tone muscles.

Pilates Ball: A small inflatable ball that can be used for support and stability during specific exercises.

Pilates Reformer: A specialized piece of equipment commonly used in Pilates studios, featuring a moving carriage and various springs to provide resistance for exercises.

Plank: A core-strengthening exercise in which you hold a push-up position with your arms extended and your body in a straight line.

Flexibility: The range of motion in your joints and muscles, which can be improved through stretching exercises.

Deep Breathing: A fundamental aspect of Pilates, involving conscious, controlled breaths to facilitate movement and relaxation.

Savasana (Corpse Pose): A relaxation pose in which you lie on your back, fully relaxed, focusing on your breath and letting go of tension.

Appendix: Additional Resources

Here are some recommended books and websites for further learning and exploration of Pilates:

Books:

Rael Isacowitz and Karen Clippinger's "Pilates Anatomy"

"The Pilates Body: The Ultimate At-Home Guide to Strengthening, Lengthening, and Toning Your Body-Without Machines" was written by Brooke Siler.

Websites:

Pilates Method Alliance: Offers information on Pilates certification, education, and resources.

Pilates Anytime: Provides a wide range of online Pilates classes for all levels.

Appendix: Index

This index provides a quick reference guide to key topics and terms covered in this guide:

Breathing: See "Deep Breathing"

Core: See "Core"

Flexibility: See "Flexibility"

Pilates Ball: See "Pilates Ball"

Pilates Mat: See "Pilates Mat"

Pilates Reformer: See "Pilates Reformer"

Plank: See "Plank"

Savasana (Corpse Pose): See "Savasana (Corpse Pose)"

Resistance Bands: See "Resistance Bands"

This appendix serves as a valuable reference section, providing you with a sample weekly routine, a glossary of key terms, and additional resources to support your Morning Pilates journey. Use it to enhance your understanding of Pilates and to further tailor your practice to your specific needs and preferences.

Appendix: Glossary

This glossary provides detailed explanations of key terms and phrases commonly used in Pilates to help you better understand the practice and its principles.

Core: The central part of the body, including the muscles of the abdomen, lower back, and pelvis. What is essential for stability is core strenght, balance, and posture. Many Pilates exercises focus on strengthening the core.

Pilates Mat: A specialized mat designed for Pilates exercises. It typically provides cushioning and a non-slip surface to ensure comfort and safety during workouts performed on the floor.

Resistance Bands: Elastic bands used in Pilates to add resistance to various exercises. They come in different strengths and can be incorporated to increase the challenge and intensity of exercises.

Pilates Ball: A small inflatable ball that is sometimes used in Pilates exercises. It can provide support, stability, and an added challenge to certain movements, particularly those targeting the core and balance.

Pilates Reformer: A piece of specialized Pilates equipment commonly found in Pilates studios. The reformer features a moving carriage connected to springs that provide variable resistance. It allows for a wide range of exercises, including those that enhance strength, flexibility, and balance.

Plank: A core-strengthening exercise in which you hold a push-up position with your arms extended and your body in a straight line from head to heels. Planks are excellent for developing core stability and strength.

Flexibility: refers to your joints' and muscles' range of motion. In Pilates, flexibility is improved through stretching exercises, helping to increase mobility and reduce the risk of injury.

Deep Breathing: A fundamental aspect of Pilates, involving conscious, controlled breaths. Deep breathing is synchronized with movements and is used to facilitate proper engagement of muscles, enhance oxygenation, and promote relaxation.

Savasana (Corpse Pose): A relaxation pose in which you lie on your back with your legs extended and your arms by your sides, palms facing up. Savasana is used in yoga and Pilates to promote relaxation, mindfulness, and a sense of calm. It allows for a deep release of tension.

Dynamic Movement: Exercises that involve controlled and deliberate movement, often focusing on fluidity and precision. Dynamic movements are a core component of Pilates, helping to build strength, coordination, and body awareness.

Isometric Contraction: A type of muscle contraction in which the muscle remains the same length while generating force. Isometric contractions are used in Pilates exercises to stabilize the core and other muscle groups.

Neutral Spine: The optimal alignment of the spine that maintains its natural curves. In Pilates, maintaining a neutral spine is emphasized to promote proper posture and minimize the risk of injury.

Mind-Body Connection: The awareness and connection between the mind and body, which is central to Pilates. It involves focusing on movements with intention and precision, enhancing concentration, and promoting mindfulness.

Pilates Principles: The foundational principles of Pilates, including concentration, control, centering, precision, breath, and flow. These principles guide the practice and ensure its effectiveness.

Matwork: A term used to describe Pilates exercises performed on a mat, typically without the use of specialized equipment like the reformer. Matwork exercises are designed to improve core strength, flexibility, and overall body conditioning.

Cadillac: A piece of Pilates equipment that provides a range of exercises, including those that emphasize stretching, flexibility, and gentle movements. The Cadillac is often used for rehabilitation and therapeutic purposes.

Joseph Pilates: The founder of the Pilates method, Joseph Pilates developed the system in the early 20th century. His principles and exercises form the basis of modern Pilates practice.

This expanded glossary provides a comprehensive understanding of essential Pilates terminology. Use it as a reference to enhance your knowledge of Pilates principles and techniques as you continue your Morning Pilates journey.

Appendix: Additional Resources

Enhance your Morning Pilates journey with these recommended resources, including books, websites, and online platforms dedicated to Pilates, fitness, and well-being.

Books:

"Anatomy of pilates" by Rael Isacowitz and Karen Clippinger

This comprehensive guide delves into the anatomy of Pilates exercises, helping you understand how each movement benefits your body.

The Pilates Body: Brooke Siler's "The Ultimate At-Home Guide to Strengthening, Lengthening, and Toning Your Body- Without Machines"

An accessible book for beginners, offering insights into Pilates fundamentals and step-by-step instructions for various exercises.

"Return to Life through Contrology" by Joseph Pilates Explore the original writings of Joseph Pilates, the founder of the Pilates method. This book provides a glimpse into his philosophy and principles.

"The Pilates Healing Bible: Tone Your Body with This Gentle, Effective Exercise System" by Melissa Cosby was published in 2008.

A practical guide that combines Pilates exercises with holistic wellness approaches, emphasizing the mind-body connection.

Websites:

Pilates Method Alliance:

The official website of the Pilates Method Alliance (PMA), providing information on Pilates certification, education, and resources. You can find certified Pilates instructors and learn about professional development opportunities.

Pilates Anytime:

An online platform offering a wide range of Pilates classes for all levels, including beginner-friendly sessions. Accessible from the comfort of your home, it allows you to practice Pilates anytime, anywhere.

Pilatesology:

A subscription-based website that features a vast library of classical Pilates workouts and tutorials. Pilatesology offers a deep dive into the traditional Pilates method.

The Balanced Life:

Created by certified Pilates instructor Robin Long, this website offers Pilates workouts and wellness resources. It's known for its emphasis on promoting a balanced and healthy lifestyle.

Online Platforms:

YouTube:

YouTube is a treasure trove of Pilates workout videos. Many certified instructors and fitness enthusiasts share free Pilates routines suitable for various levels of experience.

Gaia: Gaia is a streaming platform that offers a diverse range of Pilates and yoga classes, as well as mindfulness and wellness content. It's an excellent resource for holistic well-being.

Daily Burn:

Daily Burn provides a variety of fitness programs, including Pilates workouts. It offers both live and on-demand classes to keep your routine fresh.

Peloton:

Peloton offers live and on-demand Pilates classes through its app, along with other fitness disciplines. You can choose from a variety of instructors and class lengths.

Whether you're looking for in-depth Pilates instruction, wellness guidance, or online classes, these resources cater to various preferences and fitness levels. Explore and leverage these tools to enrich your Morning Pilates practice and nurture your well-being.

Appendix: Index

This index serves as a handy reference guide to quickly find and revisit specific topics, terms, and exercises covered in your Morning Pilates for Beginners guide.

Breathing: See "Deep Breathing"

Cadillac: See "Pilates Cadillac"

Core: See "Core"

Deep Breathing: Explanation of controlled breaths in Pilates (Page [X]).

Dynamic Movement: Exercises with controlled and deliberate motion (Page [X]).

Flexibility: Range of motion in joints and muscles (Page [X]).

Isometric Contraction: Muscle contraction where muscle length remains the same (Page [X]).

Joseph Pilates: Founder of the Pilates method (Page [X]).

Matwork: Pilates exercises performed on a mat (Page [X]).

Mind-Body Connection: Awareness and connection between mind and body (Page [X]).

Pilates Anatomy: Book by Rael Isacowitz and Karen Clippinger (Page [X]).

Pilates Anytime: Online platform for Pilates classes (Page [X]).

Pilates Ball: Small inflatable ball used in Pilates exercises (Page [X]).

Pilates Body, the: Book by Brooke Siler (Page [X]).

Pilates Mat: Specialized mat for Pilates exercises (Page [X]).

Pilates Method Alliance: Official website for Pilates resources (Page [X]).

Pilates Reformer: Specialized Pilates equipment (Page [X]).

Plank: Core-strengthening exercise (Page [X]).

Resistance Bands: Elastic bands for added resistance in Pilates (Page [X]).

Savasana (Corpse Pose): Relaxation pose in Pilates (Page [X]).

Seated Forward Bend: Stretching exercise (Page [X]).

Synchronized Breath: Breath coordinated with movement (Page [X]).

The Balanced Life: Website for Pilates workouts and wellness resources (Page [X]).

The Pilates Healing Bible: Book by Melissa Cosby (Page [X]).

Return to Life Through Contrology: Book by Joseph Pilates (Page [X]).

YouTube: Online platform for Pilates workout videos (Page [X]).

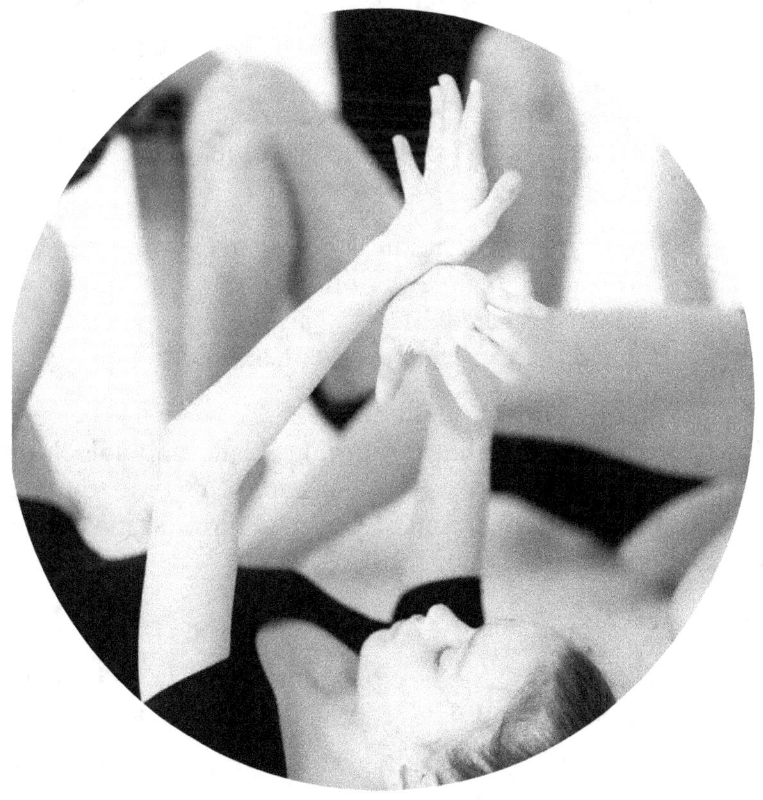

Empower Your Mornings with Pilates

As we conclude this comprehensive guide to Morning Pilates for beginners, it's time to reflect on the transformative potential of this practice and how it can positively shape your life. You've embarked on a journey that encompasses not only physical fitness but also mental clarity, balance, and a profound connection between your mind and body.

Throughout these pages, you've discovered the principles of Pilates, from mastering core strength to achieving flexibility and nurturing mindfulness. You've learned to engage in deep, purposeful breaths, synchronize them with your movements, and witnessed the incredible impact it can have on your well-being.

Pilates is more than just a morning routine; it's a commitment to self-care, a promise to prioritize your health, and a pathway to an enriched life. It's about the joy of every stretch, the strength in every movement, and the clarity in every breath.

Now, the power to embrace Morning Pilates and unlock its countless benefits is firmly in your hands. It's time to make a choice, a choice that could redefine your mornings, your days, and ultimately, your life.

Embrace Your Morning Pilates Journey

1. **Set a Start Date**: Decide on the date you'll kicks tart your Morning Pilates routine. Be committed to what you have written down

2. **Create Your Space**: Prepare a dedicated space for your practice, whether it's a corner of your living room or a serene spot in your backyard.

3. **Gather Your Resources**: Collect any equipment you'll need, such as a Pilates mat, resistance bands, or a Pilates ball.

4. **Choose Your Resources**: Explore the recommended books, websites, and online platforms in the "Additional Resources" section to expand your Pilates knowledge and access guided classes.

5. **Plan Your Routine**: Customize your weekly routine based on your goals and preferences, using the sample routine provided as a starting point.

6. **Stay Committed**: Remember that consistency is the key to success. Commit to your practice, even on days when motivation wanes.

7. **Celebrate Your Progress**: Embrace the journey, acknowledge your achievements, and celebrate every step forward.

Your mornings are a canvas, and with Morning Pilates, you have the power to paint them with vitality, strength, and inner harmony. The choice is yours, and the opportunity is here, waiting for you to seize it.

Are you ready to awaken your potential, to sculpt a stronger, more flexible body, and to embrace the serenity that comes from mind-body synergy? The time is now. Your Morning Pilates for beginner's journey awaits you. Embrace it, empower yourself, and let each morning be a testament to your dedication to a healthier, happier you.